Did I Kill My BROTHER?

The Story of the Last Three Years of the

Life of Rod Bell

AND

About My Mom

The Story of Ruby Bell's Last Fight

JEFF BELL

ISBN 978-1-0980-8653-4 (paperback)
ISBN 978-1-0980-8654-1 (digital)

Christian Faith Publishing, Inc.
832 Park Avenue
Meadville, PA 16335
www.christianfaithpublishing.com

Printed in the United States of America

ACKNOWLEDGMENTS

I want to dedicate this book to a number of people who eased the pain of my brother, my family, and my mom.

Terry Miller was the best friend my brother ever had and a real help to our family in time of need. I am sure he is a wonderful pastor down in Long Beach, California.

Dr. Heidi Beery is a true Christian doctor who shows patience, concern, and a thorough interest in her patients. We are proud to say that she is our doctor.

Melinda Gapinski was the most caring nurse in the nursing home where my brother lived for just under three years. She went out of her way to converse with Rod and meet his needs. Even now, she is still interested in our family.

Antonina and Daniel Disney owned and operated the adult foster care home where my mom stayed over eight months. In that place, there was a lot more individual attention paid to the patients, and it was a family atmosphere which my mom could thrive in. They also had a spiritual bent in their home.

Brenda and Denny Kaneshiro took over when the Disneys went on an extended vacation. They loved to pray with my mom and took special concern for her. They exemplified compassion.

Tim and Linda Bell, my brother and sister-in-law really played an important role in my mom's last days. Tim came to be with my mom and my family for five days during the last few days of her life. Linda was taking care of a major project almost all by herself so Tim could come. Her parents were moving that same week. It was a very tough job to handle on her own. She would have loved to come to help with my mom otherwise.

Livi Bell, my wife, traveled the same road I did with my brother and my mom. She often had to be my strength and guide. I know she loved them as her own family. I praise God for her.

INTRODUCTION

Sometimes in our lives, after we have gone through a tremendous struggle, we look back and are amazed that we made it through. I remember all the work I put forth in my education, and I know I would not want to go through it again; in fact, I don't think I would be able to go through it again.

My experiences with my brother dying and my mom getting Lewy body dementia are two experiences that I would never want to go through again. It was absolutely like going through hell. However, as I examine what happened during those days, there were some good things that I went through as well. I believe it made me more compassionate and more self-analyzing. I could better see what kind of man I am. It is not all nice to see. I have some pretty bad traits. When I compare them to Jesus, I see how helpless I am without Him and His forgiveness.

My attempt is to be helpful to everyone. I can help those who have gone through similar situations try to analyze themselves and maybe see how they could do a better job the next time they go through those types of experiences. In fact, I can help myself in this way as well.

I can help those who have never gone through this type of situation get an inkling of what it will be like. I have included a lot of helpful and practical things I found out that would have been nice for me to know in advance.

For those who have never gone through anything like my experience, there are two types of people: those who will go through these types of experiences and those who never will. Even if they will never go through such an experience, they can help others who find themselves experiencing a rough situation with a loved one. In all these ways, I would like to think my book will be helpful.

Even if it is just a sad commentary on life in this sinful world, it can help us see the way Jesus sees things. He didn't have to get involved and suffer with all of us who are stuck in our human situation. But He loves us so much that not only did He identify with us but also He actually became one of us and felt every horrible thing we can experience and much worse because He became sin for us on the cross. I hope this love that Jesus has for us comes out in this book in full force. That is certainly my prayer.

Although this book is written with the perspective of a Christian, I believe it can also be helpful for anyone no matter what perspective they have. This is because we are all humans, and we all suffer in one degree or another.

I hope that everybody can get a blessing from this book.

The first section of the book was written well after the events of that section took place. However, the second section of the book was written more like a journal—as it happened in general. This causes a little disjoining; the story is not over and has to be picked up later in the book. Because of this fact, I have attempted to finish every thread of the story either in another place in the body of the book or in the last chapter entitled "Tying Up Loose Ends."

My hope is that all can follow all the stories. The attempt to follow all the stories, I believe, is well worth it.

SECTION 1

Did I Kill My Brother?

CHAPTER 1

Desires Don't Always Get Met

All I wanted to do was to hold him. He had calmed my fears over fifty years ago, and I really wanted to pay him back. I remember that one night I was afraid for some reason. Who knows or remembers why? It's just one of those things you feel when you are about five years old. I don't know if I told him I was afraid, or it's just something big brothers can sense. He had come a long way in his concern for me. When I was a baby, he used to get up in the night and pee on me. I can only imagine he didn't like all the attention I was getting. But after more than four years of getting used to me and actually loving me, Rod felt sorry that I was scared.

We both felt it was later than it really was. It had seemed to me that I could not sleep for hours. However, when Rod got up to see what time it was, it was only about 8:00 p.m. After a while, I had calmed down, and he went back to his bed to sleep. I would never forget that experience.

Now, it was my turn to pay him back for his love he showed over fifty years ago and ever since. My older brother, Rod, was not in good health. His life was one of pain and misery. He had had diabetes since he was about twenty. He had also fallen off a scaffold working construction. He had serious back problems and was in constant pain. He had had many girlfriends and even a wife once. His stepdaughter was the apple of his eye, but that ended when her mother divorced Rod. He missed that little girl so. At this point in his life, he felt he had nothing to offer a woman, and perhaps, he was right. However, he still had great love for others. He exemplified a Christian in that respect even though he did not claim to be one.

He had lost a leg by amputation due to complications from his diabetes. I loved him, but I felt he was not too lovable to most people, and he was the type of person most people would not want to get too close to. I felt sorry for him. He had a promising future when he was young—good looking, in good shape, he easily made friends, and made a good living in construction. But now he didn't seem to have much of a life. Oh, how I wanted to crawl up in bed with him and hold him. He could feel loved. He deserved it because he loved me and my family (my wife, Livi, and two girls, Janet and Crystal) very much. He deserved it as someone who Jesus died for. However, by the time I figured out what I should do and what I knew he would love, he got a case of MERSA (a skin infection that was easily contracted and was dangerous).

Now it was too late. I was hardly allowed to be with him in the same room. What a letdown. I am glad I never told him because he would have been let down too.

I was born with a handicap. My hands and arms were badly deformed. I have gone through many difficult times in my life. When I was very young, other children would make fun of me. Once, when in kindergarten, I walked from home as usual but did not go all the way to school. I was afraid of the other children saying something mean to me again. I stayed by the railroad tracks to wait until the other children got out of school, and then I would go home. Being so young, I did not realize that the tracks were close by the school, and anybody at the school could see me. Much to my surprise, my mom soon came. The school had called her to report that I was waiting by the tracks.

My mom loved me. I knew it. I did not get into any trouble from my mom. However, in my family, it was my dad that we had to fear. When he came home, we might get a whipping with a stick he cut off a bush just outside our bedroom window. But that night was different. My dad said something I will never forget. He said, "Jeff, I wish I could have your hands and you could have mine." He told me that I would not get in trouble this time, but I had to go to school. I was in a very loving family. I thank God every day for that fact.

I don't believe that sports and competition are the best for the character of any child. If the child cannot play very well, he could be scarred for life. If he became one of the best in the school, he would have pride issues. However, for some reason, I felt that in order to be accepted in the school, I had to excel at sports. I mean every sport I could possibly play. I didn't realize it then, but my brother, Rod, did one of the most unselfish things a brother could do. In order to help me excel at most sports, he would take his recess time, and we would throw the football back and forth or throw the baseball to each other. He would also help me shoot and dribble the basketball. I began to get very good at all sports. I was soon playing with all the other children and doing at least as good as the other children. Boy, did I owe my brother my love and care. The realization didn't come until he was basically an invalid. I realized how selfish I had been.

Rod had also been my protector, putting his life on the line at least once. When both of us were walking home from school, a future gang member was bothering me. Rod told him to leave me alone and pick on someone his own size. The young man pulled a knife on Rod, and there was a standoff. The situation finally resolved after a minute or so. My brother would have given his life for me.

It was my turn to take care of him. My wife, Livi, and I would meet him at doctor's appointments and buy supplies for him to supplement the care he received in the nursing home. Livi was his caregiver, and I was his accountant. He trusted me to be his power of attorney, and I took the responsibility seriously. I was glad to take that responsibility from him. He could concentrate on other things in life now that I was taking care of things on the financial end.

Rod had four nieces that meant the world to him. He loved all of them very much and was interested in all their activities. He was not able to attend many of the activities of my daughters near the end of his life because he couldn't get around well and was constantly in pain. Since he lived near us in Oregon, he could not attend any of the activities of my brother, Tim, and his wife, Linda, and their two girls, Melissa and Stephanie who live in Southern California. He really felt bad when Tim's oldest daughter, Melissa, got married, and he could not go. I felt bad that Rod was not involved. At Tim's house, we did talk with Rod on the phone once. Unfortunately, Melissa was not available to talk. She was on her honeymoon.

A very touching occasion was when he was able to see his first grandnephew. Rod was not doing well at all, but he was all smiles—the love showed. It is a terrible thing when people have to live in a nursing home, and people only visit them for just a few minutes or so. It feels like it is just out of duty. I would have liked to spend hours with him seeing my grandson. However, I know it was a long trip for my daughter, Crystal, and her husband, Mike, especially with a five-month-old. I know they loved Rod very much.

I don't want to make a savior out of my brother, but there are several similarities in our relationship. At times, I felt I was helping him out of duty. Sometimes, we know we ought to obey Jesus, but we are doing it because we know we should, and we don't want to be lost. It is not really out of love for Him. At times, it was a burden to help Rod. Sometimes, he was antagonistic toward the doctors he went to see or the caregivers and dieticians who worked in the nursing home. It was hard to smooth things over when he was upset and swearing at them. He wanted to help many people, but he could not stand to be treated badly or taken advantage of. His understanding of what was good for him was not very good, and he disagreed with most professionals about his care. I blamed the diabetes for that because I want to think the best of Rod.

There was also a long period of time when Rod entered the nursing home that I had to deal with all his stuff. To most people, it was junk. But I knew what most of it was because I had grown up with him, and I felt that some of it was quite valuable. In fact, at this time, I am still trying to sell much of it. Because I was spending a lot of time going through his stuff and finding places for everything and putting up shelves in the 10x20 storage unit with the help of a good man and now friend Larry Smith and his wife, Carol (who recently passed away), I really didn't have time to see Rod too much. I would have liked to spend at least an hour a day, but sometimes, I could only spend about forty-five minutes. I had a family I wanted to spend time with also. Sometimes, I didn't have time to visit him at all. I would also bring stuff to the nursing home for Rod to see if he would throw anything away or try to sell it. I think he remembered just about everything he had, which was an amazing feat in itself. It was with great thought and trouble that he was willing to part with anything.

If I would look back on my life and how Rod was there for me and loved me, I could help him out of love because he first loved me. That is how it is with Jesus. He first loved us. We didn't deserve it, but He was in extreme love with us. That is really the only way we can obey Him. The power is in the love. Over time, I learned by experience to do for Rod out of love.

I felt sorry for Rod and wanted to make his life have meaning. I felt really badly when he was not taken care of. There was a nurse at the nursing home named Melinda Gapinski that I could really tell cared for him and was interested in his life and stories. He loved to cheer people up with his jokes although they were shady a lot of the time. He was lonely, and he wanted people to like him and, for the most part, need him.

I have learned that our desires do not always come true. The only way our desires can help a person, if they are actually the best thing for them, is for us to carry them out at some time. My desire to hold Rod, if never carried out, could never help him. However, that unfulfilled desire could actually benefit me whether carried out or not. We can gain an actual picture of our true self, or we can realize that we have had the heart of God placed inside us—at least until we drive Him away again. But when we send Him out, He is knocking on the door of our hearts again. He will not give up easily. To have the heart of God placed inside of us is a tremendous privilege that everyone has the opportunity to have if we accept Jesus into our hearts.

CHAPTER 2

Three Attitudes Toward
the Incapacitated

I have discovered that different people react differently to loved ones that are so sick they cannot function physically, mentally, or emotionally. I have also discovered that I cannot really judge people for the way they react. It is simply the way they can deal with the horrible, almost impossible, situation they are dealing with.

One way people react toward their loved ones that cannot function is to put up a wall between their loved one and themselves. They don't pay much attention to them because they hurt so much and, frankly, do not know how to act around them. It is most likely the result of a lack of maturity or a lack of experience. They can also be fearful that they say the wrong thing or do the wrong thing. The last thing they would want to do is to hurt someone's feelings or hurt them physically by incorrectly helping them get up or lie down or something.

I remember when I had my first fulltime job. A coworker lost her mother. The coworker was in her fifties and had been very nice and helpful to me in my life. I felt like I needed to go to her house and comfort her, but I had no idea what to do to comfort her. I was fearful to hurt her feelings or make her feel worse. I ended up going and struggling through the situation.

I just told her I was sorry for her and her family. She took over from there, thanking me and telling me about her mother and how much she loved and missed her.

Because of that experience, I learned better how to deal with those types of situations. It is good to just act on what you know to be right, but I can't blame somebody for not following through. After all, it is possible to hurt somebody's feelings by saying or doing the wrong thing.

Another type of reaction is a little more helpful. We can care for them mechanically by not showing the love and concern that is best to show.

The third type of reaction to the extremely needy loved one is to care for them with love and patience. I have found in my experience that in order to really love and care for them, you must suffer with them. This, of course, is a very difficult task. You can start out doing it and get lost because it is too painful. Then you fall back to, at the least, the second reaction.

I believe that in order to keep suffering with your loved one, you need a godly love placed in your heart by none other than God Himself. He has promised this and is certainly able to keep His promises. And another thing is, if you hurt someone's feelings, you can always say you are sorry. It could be worth the try.

CHAPTER 3

A Time When Rod Wasn't in Our Lives (Learn from His Stuff)

There was a period of time when Rod did not have much contact with our family. I am not sure how long this was, but it was at least twelve years. We knew he was off doing things that our family did not approve of. In this aspect, Rod was like the prodigal son in the Bible. He had some friends that were in music groups that he hung around with. He also spent much time trying to imitate Kenny Loggins and trying to meet him or have him do songs that Rod wrote. My brother, Tim, and I were actually too busy to follow what he was doing. We were getting our education and getting our first jobs. I know that, at least, I was also very selfish and did not, like the older brother of the prodigal, go out to find him. He had hurt our parents and (I'll speak for myself) I really was not too pleased with him.

There was a lot going on in Rod's life that we didn't have a clue about. From the outside, it seemed like a lot of silliness. During this time, he had fallen from the scaffold and was injured beyond repair—even though the doctors originally gave him the green light to continue working.

He was getting continuously worse and incapable of working. He was also building up a line of thinking that made God seem like an unjust being. This would eventually lead me to not want to discuss religion with him. The words that came out of his mouth were very blasphemous, and I could not bear to hear them. I was actually scared to get into a conversation with him. My mom felt the same way.

It is sad, but there were so many things I didn't find out about Rod until he passed away. This is to my shame.

One awakening of Rod's missing life was during the memorial service held at the nursing home where he lived out the last years of his life. The pastor who officiated the service was Terry Miller. He had been a guitar player and singer in a local rock band in Southern California. Now he is a pastor. He had been Rod's best friend for many years. He really loved Rod and tried to help him many times. He wrote a letter supporting Rod in getting Social Security Disability. My dad went to bat for Rod several times to finally get the settlement and used Terry's letter to help provide proof of Rod's frames of mind. Terry had tried to get Rod to be involved with some money-making projects for Rod to make some money. But Rod had little interest in doing any of these because he didn't want to ruin the chances for the others involved. Rod had very little self-confidence after the fall, and the diabetes started taking him down.

Terry painted a picture of Rod that I had never heard before. He said that Rod was the best friend he ever had and that he would help Terry with ideas for the concerts that were very amusing. Rod had the idea of putting a blow dryer on some handle bars to blow Terry's long hair while he was performing a song about a motorcyclist running down the highway with his hair blowing in the wind. He shared other stories as well.

Terry had given his heart to Jesus later in his life, and Rod was supportive but never gave his heart to Jesus that anyone knows about. Terry was very sad about that. Rod had always been supportive of Terry's children, encouraging them in their endeavors and their failures. Rod had been a true Christian to many people without being a true Christian on the surface. That gave Terry hope and also gave me hope as well.

Another way I learned a lot about Rod was by going through his junk. Rod was a true hoarder. He had his bedroom at my mom's house full of stuff. It was the same with the garage, which had many shelves, trunks, tables, and stacked boxes full of junk. Well, I learned that although much of it was stuff I would never have been attracted to (like the collection of the two metal ends of cardboard frozen juice containers), a lot of it was valuable and interesting, at least to me. I found that Rod was a genius in many areas; some are areas I never knew existed.

Rod was a veritable electronics genius. He made detailed schematics of projects he had made in his bedroom or that he planned to make some day when he could muster up the patience, strength, and/or ability to do so.

Some of the areas Rod had researched were astronomy (including alien beings), history, geography, science, natural medicine, actors, politicians, natural household cleaning solutions and, of course, electronics. He even saved an internet article on how to make an atomic bomb. He had a massive cassette tape collection, some of which he called "car tunes" which he carried in his Toyota minivan. Of course, they were all well categorized and itemized on several lists. He also had hundreds of VHS video tapes with movies, TV programs, and home videos. I have been trying to sell them along with several music collections ever since Rod passed away. I finally did sell them at a great loss. I am glad I didn't pay for them all.

From Rod's passion for Kenny Loggins, I finally sold quite a collection of records, tapes, 8-tracks, CDs, video tapes, and a pamphlet about Kenny Loggins's book. I sold a jacket that Rod had that looked like one that Kenny had.

I also found and read some letters that brought out some of the grief and pain that Rod went through as well as his attempts to try to help Terry Miller's son, TJ. I found documents sent to Social Security that my father wrote to try to get Rod a settlement. I found out that Rod was extremely depressed most of the time, and his outlet for relief was trying to help others. That was a wonderful quality and skill he had.

I found a letter from TJ thanking Rod for all his support in his life. I also found a letter from Rod that he sent with a check to help with an operation that a very young girl needed to have in order to live. He cared about so many people. I was so proud of him.

My greatest prize was a suicide letter that Rod wrote in the event that his attempt worked. He basically told everyone that he loved them. It was especially heartwarming what he wrote about and to Terry. He had attempted suicide several times in his life. I knew about a couple of them. This time he was going to just give up and die. It was a type of mind-over-matter attempt. Rod really believed that he had this kind of power. He said he used it to control his pain on several occasions. Of course, all of them failed, and I thank God about that.

The moral of the story is that a person's junk tells a lot about them. However, to know these things about them first-hand is much, much, better. My hope is that many will learn from my mistakes.

CHAPTER 4

Doctors, Doctors, Doctors

My brother didn't have a lot of respect for doctors. They had to earn his respect and, in his eyes, very few of them did. He thought he knew everything about diabetes and would argue vehemently with any doctor who didn't agree with him. If they had the attitude that they knew everything about his case, he didn't have much good to say about them.

He even argued with the specialist who was training him on the insulin pump, which he desired to have for many years. He thought it would be the end of his problems because he thought he could live a normal life. It was designed to help with that, but it did not cure diabetes. He wanted to eat anything he wanted whenever he wanted. This included eating ice cream late at night or early in the morning. He had strange habits and strange hours. Nothing in his life was on a regular schedule, which is important for diabetics. This made for many fights with the specialist and other doctors who, he thought, wanted to control his life just to put him in his place. I felt sorry for most of the doctors, but some may have kind of deserved it because of their "better than you" attitude. Rod particularly hated that all his problems were linked to his diabetes according to most of the doctors. He felt it was just laziness—not wanting to look into everything thoroughly because they figured he was beyond help.

There was one doctor who was much different. It happened to be Rod's primary care physician. He did argue with her a little, but she actually earned his respect because she actually listened to him and really cared about him. My wife and I have always been impressed with her. She is Dr. Heidi Beery. She worked with Rod as much as anyone could and was always patient with him. She is a Christian, and it shows. People can really tell that she wants to make a difference in Roseburg. She is even involved in a program to teach people how to live a healthier lifestyle. My wife and I have actually been following this healthy lifestyle for about twenty-seven years, advancing in our understanding as we learn.

We all prized her as we went through the stages of Rod's final years. At the time of this writing, my wife and I are very fortunate to have her as our primary care physician. It is so nice to have a doctor who you know is on your side and patient with her patients.

CHAPTER 5

Did I Kill Him?

This chapter could either be seen as providential or as bad luck depending on how I look at it. It is the hardest chapter to write because it drums up old emotions of the hardest part of my life to that point.

I had been advised to sign myself up as Rod's medical power of attorney. I already had power of attorney for his finances, but the administration of the nursing home thought somebody should be able to direct his care. He might not be able to respond to direct his own.

I remember calling around to find a notary who could come to Rod's room and sign me up. It could have been Thursday, but I think it was Friday that the lady came. Rod signed it, and I signed it, and the lady signed it. I might have needed a signature of a witness as well. It seemed very unimportant at the time.

Little did I know that we would need to put it into action the very next day (Saturday). We were at church and received a call that Rod was acting strange. He seemed to be almost in a coma, and his blood sugar was extremely high. He refused to be taken to the hospital or be helped in any way. They wanted us to come and try to convince him that he needed to go to the hospital.

It was not an easy task to get him to go to the hospital. In fact, he still refused. It was like he didn't believe that he had an urgent problem. I didn't want to go against his wishes, but I was afraid staying at the nursing home would make his health deteriorate more. He had been through similar situations before and always come out of it—either by going to the hospital or by doing basically nothing. After all, he felt he could control his blood sugar and other bodily conditions by placing his mind over his matter.

Livi convinced me that Rod needed to go to the hospital. He was really upset about it, and I felt bad that he was upset with me, but I felt it was the best solution. The ambulance came and took him to the emergency room of the hospital. The events that transpired did not help my dilemma of uncertainty about taking him there.

I remember the doctor asking Rod many questions to see if he was with it or not. He seemed to be able to answer all the questions. Then he asked Rod if he knew who the man was next to him (which was me). Rod answered, "Jeffrey Charles Bell." Then they asked him if he knew where he was. He answered, "Jeffrey Charles Bell." I don't remember if they asked him another question, but if they did, he answered "Jeffrey Charles Bell" again. I really don't think he was mixed up. I believe he was mad at me.

The next thing that happened was they wanted to put a catheter in. Livi and I left the room, and that was an experience I will never forget. Through the door, we heard Rod screaming because of the pain. I don't remember if I cried or just felt like it. Oh, how could I have done this to him? Maybe I should have just let him stay at the nursing home. Maybe he would have been alright and spared all the pain and inconvenience.

After Rod was admitted and having his blood sugar regulated, he was really out of it and basically sleeping. We went home that night and prayed for his recovery. I had done enough, really.

On Sunday, I went and visited Rod, and he seemed much improved. We were talking like brothers again. I thought he was well on his way to recovery like so many times before. After a couple of hours, I went home again, feeling pretty good about the situation.

Either that night or the next morning, my whole family came down with the worst flu we had ever had. We couldn't do anything. We just sat around. Our good friend Brandtley came over and made vegetable smoothies to help us gain our strength. We stayed home that day. The next day, we felt like staying home again because we were still a little weak. However, in the early afternoon, we received a very shocking phone call. The nurse at the hospital told us we better come quickly to see Rod because they didn't know if he would make it through the night.

"How is that?" I asked. The last time I saw him, he had been so much improved. They told me he had contracted a very powerful flu virus, and it had gone into pneumonia, and his lungs were filling with fluids. Apparently, he had the same flu we did, but his immune system was very compromised. Also, he had taken so many antibiotics in his life that no antibiotics would work on this. I will never know if he contracted the virus in the hospital or from us or from the nursing home. So you can see that I am not sure I did the right thing. So my getting the health power of attorney could have been providential or could have been the worst luck I ever had.

We went to see Rod, and he was not able to talk with us. He was basically in a coma with an oxygen mask on to help him get enough oxygen. He had told me before to never let them put that mask on again because it suffocated him. Here he was with it on again. What should I do?

The doctor on duty for Rod was a very nice Christian woman. She took us to a private area and talked with us. She told us how both lungs had filled up with fluid extremely quickly. There was nothing they could do except keep him on oxygen and give him morphine to ease the pain.

Livi had to leave because of work, but my mom and I stayed. We watched him trying to remove the mask because it really bothered him. We tried to tell him that the mask was the only thing that was keeping him alive, but he kept on fighting it. What was really happening was that he could not get enough oxygen to feel comfortable because of the pneumonia. He thought it was because of the mask. With our approval, they gave him more morphine so he would not fight the mask, then the breathing machine could work efficiently.

I remember that God worked out that Rod became aware at one point. He reached up with one of his hands and opened his right eye so he could see us. We tried to communicate with him and think we actually succeeded. My mom had a brilliant idea. She suggested we say the Lord's Prayer as we did every night when we were little when my mom put us to bed. We recited it and then told Rod "good night" for the last time ever. Since Rod was not a proclaimed Christian, we hope this prayer would wake him up to his need of the Savior. Oh, how I hope it did.

I remember Rod's oxygen level dropped down into the seventies. The nurse asked if there were any relatives and friends they should call. I told them to call my brother, Tim, and my daughter, Janet. My daughter came, and my brother and his wife called. While they were talking with us, Rod's oxygen level went way down, and I thought it was the end. I cried to my brother, "This is horrible, I got to go. Rod is dying." Well, as so many times before, Rod rebounded, and his oxygen levels went back up. My mom and I decided we could do no more good there, and I took her home, and I went home expecting any time to get "that" phone call.

I think it was about six in the morning that the phone call came. They told us we should get there to view the body as soon as possible because the undertaker people were scheduled to pick up the body. I called my brother and my mom and told them the news. My brother lives in California and could not come, of course. My mom didn't want to come. She had been through enough, me too, actually.

I dropped Janet and Livi off at the entrance and parked the car. When I got to the room, I could hear them crying in the room. I entered and immediately started crying out loud, uncontrollably. They had Rod fixed up nicely. I was very thankful for that since the people at the hospital where my dad died had done nothing for him. My dad looked like someone in a Halloween movie.

We cried and talked for about twenty minutes, with Rod's body in the room, and then let the men take him on a gurney. I remember thinking to myself, *Did I kill my brother?*

I understand that this is a fairly normal thought when somebody's medical care was under your direction. After going over things, I realized in my mind that I did the right thing, even though he died. However, emotionally, I still have not fully come to grips with it, even after over three years. It is getting better however. I talked with Dr. Beery a month or so after Rod's death saying, "I felt responsible for his death." She told my wife and me, "How do you think I feel every time I lose a patient. I go over and over everything I did to make sure I did the right thing." As I mentioned before, his doctor is a wonderful person who really cares about her patients and a good Christian woman.

Oh, how I miss my brother!

CHAPTER 6

This World Still Has Good People

In this violent and corrupt world, we often distrust people automatically because we see all the crimes committed by gangs, groups, and politically charged people. The outpouring of love and support our family experienced during this crisis showed us that there are still good people out there.

Of course, our church family was very supportive. Many, who didn't even know my brother, came to the memorial service. The best nurse at the nursing home where Rod lived, Melinda Gapinski, came to the service and told us how much she appreciated Rod and grieved over his death. I saw her more recently, and she again told me how much she missed Rod and how special he was.

A real shocker was that we received a very nice Christian sympathy card from the doctor on duty when Rod made a turn for the worse. She didn't even know us. Wherever I went to close Rod's business, people told me they were so sorry for our loss. Believe me, there are a lot of good people in this otherwise bad world.

It is for the reason that there are still good people in this world that I am writing this book. It is a way of thanking them and also to help them in case they have to go through something like this. Thanks to all who loved Rod and supported our family in any way. God is love.

SECTION 2

About My Mom

(Made for Honor)

CHAPTER 1

A Forgotten Commandment

There seems to be a very important commandment that, in today's world, is basically forgotten. If you look carefully, every commandment of the ten is forgotten today, but this one, if kept, would bring continuity to our society as no other one could. The text below describes the world today.

> There is a generation that curseth their father, and doth not bless their mother. There is a generation that are pure in their own eyes, and yet is not washed from their filthiness. There is a generation, O how lofty are their eyes! And their eyelids are lifted up. There is a generation, whose teeth are as swords, and their jaw teeth as knives, to devour the poor from off the earth, and the needy from among men. (Proverbs 30:11–14)

The first verse describes the reason for the rest of the verses. But it also describes the results of the rest of the verses. Of course, the commandment it is talking about is the fifth commandment which says, "Honour thy father and thy mother:

that thy days may be long upon the land which the Lord thy God giveth thee" (Exodus 20:12).

If our children do not obey the fifth commandment, they typically believe whatever they "feel is true" is right. Today our young people do not believe in absolutes. They believe that truth for their parents is not the truth for them. They see things differently than their parents do.

The problem does not stop there. This type of thinking leads the children to further dishonor their parents. Could it possibly be that their teeth will become as swords, and they will be willing to abandon their parents and even to break the next commandment, "Thou shalt not kill?" I know this "teeth as swords" metaphor usually describes a situation where they will say bitter, hurtful words against others; could it also be that when the lines are drawn between those who totally love God and keep His commandments and those who have totally thrown in their lives with Satan, the children will be on the side of those who will want to kill the true believers—their parents?

This is the danger many are in today. We see a generation who only want to satisfy their passions and fulfill their rights. They have no desire to be servants as Jesus was. Jesus didn't protest anything done to Him. He was not violent. We should not be either.

Do we see children abandoning their parents when they get old and feeble and maybe senile? I have a little bit different vantage point now. My mother is in a memory care facility. My mom's dementia is a special kind of dementia—one that, I believe, is the absolute worst kind. It is called Lewy body dementia. It is the disease, or condition, that Robin Williams had that drove him to commit suicide. Of course, the diagnosis is only based on her symptoms because I found out recently that the only way to truly diagnose Lewy body is with an autopsy.

The disease came on suddenly to us. Of course, there were most likely symptoms for years (some that she hid from us), but we didn't put it together until she started to act very differently from her sweet self. Upon looking at her stuff when my brother, sister-in-law, my wife, and I packed her up, we found a lot of books with mind teasers and games to strengthen the mind and figured that my mom knew something was wrong with her.

She was living in a retirement village and doing very well. After a few years of living there, she, all of a sudden, had some problems with what she categorized as gossip. The gossip didn't seem too serious to us, but to her, it was a great sin that she apologized for over and over again. She also started confessing to us certain things she had done during her earlier life. She got very stressed out about just about everything, and it scared us. She started saying strange things like the police were going to come and arrest her, and she had to be naked for them to take her picture for the front of the newspaper. It was very, very strange.

We took her to the emergency room a couple of times for pains and for falling, and they could not find anything wrong with her. Finally, after a bad fall, my wife got them to keep her, asking them if they were willing to be responsible if she fell and bled to death because she was on blood thinner.

Keeping my mom in the hospital was a great relief to Livi and me because we were exhausted spending our days and nights with her and basically guarding her. She would get up in the night and walk the halls of the building she lived in. We didn't get much sleep except for when it was not our turn to watch her.

She was in the hospital in a special section where the inpatients are mentally disturbed. There was a lot of screaming and crying going on, and it could only make all the patients more scared. She was there for over a week.

One of the days before my brother came into town, my mom started to exhibit another personality. Instead of being her usual genteel self, she started telling jokes much like a standup comedian. My daughter, Janet, visited, and, at first, thought my mom was a lot better. However, she soon realized something strange was happening. Thank God it only lasted one day.

When my brother and his wife came, they helped pack my mom's stuff to put in a storage unit, and then they oversaw my mom's care as Livi and I had a prior commitment that took us out of town for almost a week. When we returned, my brother and I, along with our wives, decided the best place for her was in a memory care facility. She went to a facility within a couple of days of our return, and my brother and his wife returned to their home.

It was a new life for my mom, and she might not have ever gotten used to it. It was kind of like a continuation of her stay in the hospital with all the residents acting strangely and making it a scary place to be. But what can you do?

I tried to visit my mom every day and read the Bible to her and sometimes play the piano for her. It can be a blessing, and it can be a real horrible experience.

I will share a blessing. Our family keeps the Bible Sabbath, which is Friday at sunset through Saturday at sunset. One Sabbath afternoon, our family and a friend went to play the piano for my mom. At first, she was leery about going out into the lobby. But after she got out there, it just got better and better. Our friend was playing the piano, and we were all singing old-fashioned Christian songs that we all seemed to know the words to. My mom was singing and really enjoying the spiritual time.

Then a resident named Freddy came out into the lobby and joined us. He was a very good singer. After getting through singing a song, he would shout, "Thank you, Jesus!" After a while, there were several residents out there—some singing and some just listening and enjoying.

Then my mom wanted to get up and sit on the piano bench and play the piano. She hadn't done that for many years. Of course, it brought tears of joy to our eyes. She seemed more alert than she had for a couple of months and, more importantly, more at peace. It was worth our efforts.

Do you know there are residents there—many of them—that I have never seen a loved one come to spend time with them? A caregiver told Livi that many of them have no family come to see them on a regular basis. This could possibly be the result of this generation thinking they are wise and wanting everything just for themselves. I think I have a little of that because I sometimes understand how they feel.

The day after we played the piano for my mom, she told me that the night before, she had horrible thoughts that she was the devil, etc. I kind of expected she would be better after that wonderful experience and on the road to recovery. But it didn't happen. You get the idea that nothing you do helps the situation and have slight feelings of giving up.

The fifth commandment is a very full commandment with a lot of meaning. It shows the unselfish love that Jesus has for us. He has done everything for us, and sometimes He probably feels that nothing He does helps. I need this unselfish love, don't you? I need to take the good with the bad. I need to be encouraged by the days when my mother seems alert and interested and calm and not be dashed to the lowest dumps when she is screaming and moaning and crying and imagining the most bizarre things you can think of. In fact, most of the things she imagines, nobody would ever have thought of. Young people, you might be tempted to think your parents' views are crazy now but just wait. I need to love and care for my mother because she needs it and not because I will get anything from it. I need to be steady in my faith also and rely totally on Jesus. That is what it means to keep the fifth commandment.

However, there is a promise in the fifth commandment. It can be taken two ways, and it becomes more apparent as one goes through life. The way most people see it, "That thy days may be long upon the land which the Lord thy God giveth thee," is that you will live a long life upon the land God has given you. This also can be taken two ways: on earth or on the new earth. What a wonderful promise this is. The reward for honoring your parents is eternal life, and I really look forward to it now.

The second way it can be taken is that your days will be long enough to accomplish everything God wants you to. This lets me know that the hour or so I take to visit my mom is not going to hinder my getting everything accomplished during the day that the Lord intends me to accomplish. My family is busier than we have ever been. It keeps me awake at night just thinking about all I have to do. But God knows what has to be done and has helped in many ways.

My view of the fifth commandment has become more important as I and my mother have gotten older. It is a precious quality to love and honor your parent. You can feel that God is with you because you are doing what He wants you to do. You can also have the hope that your children will love and support you when you get into this situation. With everything going on, I sometimes feel it might not be too far away.

Now I want to shift gears and explore more dimensions of this wonderful commandment because I believe there are more dimensions.

> Especially dreadful is the thought of a child turning in hatred upon a mother who has become old and feeble, upon whom has come those infirmities of disposition attendant upon second childhood. How patiently, how tenderly, should children bear with such a mother! Tender words which will not irritate the spirit should be spoken. A true Christian will never be unkind, never under any circumstances be neglectful of his father or mother, but will heed the command, "Honour thy father and thy mother." God has said, "Thou shalt rise up before the hoary head, and honour the face of the old man." (E.G. White: The Adventist Home, p. 362–363)

> Children, let your parents, infirm and unable to care for themselves, find their last days filled with contentment, peace, and love. For Christ's sake let them go down to the grave receiving from you only words of kindness, love, mercy, and forgiveness. You desire the Lord to love and pity and forgive you, and to make all your bed in your sickness, and will you not treat others as you would wish to be treated yourself? (Ibid. p. 363)

While the parents live it should be the children's joy to honor and respect them. They should bring all the cheerfulness and sunshine into the life of the aged parents that they possibly can. They should smooth their pathway to the grave. There is no better recommendation in this world than that a child has honored his parents, no better record in the books of heaven than that he has loved and honored father and mother. (E.G. White: My Life Today, p. 278)

We find that the fifth commandment is a two-way street. It is up to the parents to teach and exemplify the fifth commandment to their children. By the way we treat our parents, we are setting an example for our children that we will benefit from in future years. We must also treat our children with love and respect so they can see how to interact with us later and with others as well.

This interaction should also extend to all the members of the family unit.

The family firm is a sacred, social society, in which each member is to act a part, each helping the other. The work of the household is to move smoothly, like the different parts of well-regulated machinery.

Every member of the family should realize that a responsibility rests upon him individually to do his part in adding to the comfort, order, and regularity of the family. One should not work against another. All should unitedly engage in the good work of encouraging one another; they should exercise gentleness, forbearance, and patience; speak in low, calm tones, shunning confusion; and each doing his utmost to lighten the burdens of the mother... (Adventist Home, p. 179)

What do you think about adopted children? Do they fall into the framework of the fifth commandment? Are they to love and be loved with never-ending godly love? I believe they do fall into that framework. I was thinking about this, and the Lord brought to my mind a good argument to prove to me that they do. Romans 8:15 states, "Ye have not received the spirit of bondage again to fear; but ye have received the Spirit of adoption, whereby we cry, Abba, Father." And Ephesians 1:5–6 says, "Having predestinated us unto the adoption of children by Jesus Christ to himself, according to the good pleasure of his will, to the praise of the glory of his grace, wherein he hath made us accepted in the beloved."

So are we God's children by birth or by adoption? Adam was called the son of God, and that is as close as any human—other than Jesus when He took our flesh—has ever been to being a child of God by birth. We can only hope to be God's son or daughter by adoption. Jesus tells us that the way to become His son or daughter or brother or sister is by hearing the word of God and doing it (Luke 8:21).

If we are going to exemplify God's love by keeping the fifth commandment, it makes sense to me that, that relationship includes our adopted children as well as our children by birth.

So we have found out that the fifth commandment calls us to honor everyone in our family. Given that Jesus said who His mother and brethren are, ought we to have honor and God's love for our fellow members of God's church as well? I believe we are to have the same love for them. We are to care for them as Jesus cares for His church. But Jesus also had love for His enemies. It is certainly a very, very high calling—one that is not possible without Jesus enthroned within.

We need to put back in place the principles of the fifth commandment in our homes and in the church and in society. What a need there is.

CHAPTER 2

Meet My Mom

If you ever met my mom, you would have thought she was the sweetest woman in the world. She was very polite and loving and kind to everyone. But she was especially kind to her children. I was one of them, and I know.

As you know, I am handicapped. I was not mentally handicapped; I was physically handicapped. But many people in the world can't separate the two. They treat everyone with a physical handicap as if they are slow or, in some way, mentally incapable. These were the type of people who were responsible for screening students into kindergarten where I went to school. They wanted to put me into the special education class. This made my mom go to work for me. She kind of bargained with them to get me into the regular classroom. She asked them, "If he can demonstrate that he can learn certain things, will you allow him into the regular classroom?" Thank God they agreed.

My mom instantly went about teaching me to learn my ABCs and numbers through one hundred which, along with colors, was most of what the students had to accomplish by the end of the year in kindergarten. I learned and demonstrated that I knew these things and was allowed to be in the regular classroom. Other than the emotional trauma mentioned before, it made my kindergarten experience easier than most of the other students. I was ahead.

My mom was very involved with all of us boys in our education but especially with me—maybe because I learned to expect her help. Before my freshman year in high school, my mom taught me quite a bit of typing because I was required to take typing. She also taught me quite a bit of shorthand before I took that. I excelled at everything she helped me with. So I was getting help in scholastic achievements from my mom and in sports from my brother Rod.

Later in life, I remember talking with my mom one night about not having any girls interested in me and feeling like I would never get married. She told me that it was possible that I wouldn't, but she would pray that the right girl would come along that was after a good man and not just for physical attributes. I believe all her prayers were answered for me, but the one I am most thankful for was for a good wife. I am very thankful for Livi, my Guatemalan sweetheart. She also is very helpful to me. God has richly blessed me with her.

Throughout the years, my mom has continued to pray for us all. She was praying for our jobs, our children, our cars, our Christian experience and who knows what else. It hurts me that this disease has taken away her social, physical, and spiritual skills, but I know God understands. I will get her mind back with me when Jesus comes again. Oh, I can't wait.

She has also helped financially to all of us children. I would have to say that we would not be living in our country home if it were not for her help. Even now, she feels guilty because she did not help her children enough. I try to let her know that she has given more to her children than any three other mothers. She sometimes gets it.

CHAPTER 3

Little Glimpses of Her Self

My mom seems to travel in phases emotionally. Some days, she is really bad, and other days, she isn't as bad. A very few days, she is good. But she is never great.

One day, I was visiting my mom, and she was crying as usual. I was praying for her more than usual during my visit. I usually come in and think I have a lot to tell her, but with no or little input from her, the conversation doesn't last very long. She was crying seemingly more continuously than usual. I thought to myself, *What am I going to do?* I had used up my arsenal of secrets to comfort her.

Then I noticed that her crying was actually to the tune of "For Those Tears I Died." It was on a CD that I had started to play for her of my daughter, Janet, and our friend, Brandtley. What an amazing thing that was to behold. It told me there was something left spiritually inside. I praised my Lord and Savior for that little taste of what was left.

Since then, I have heard her cry-sing several times. Each time, I am amazed and thankful.

A few months before that, I had seemed to bother my mom when I visited. Livi suggested that I go visit her every other day instead of every day. Maybe it was too stressful for her for me to come every day. So now I go about every other day. Sometimes

I will go two or three days in a row if I didn't have a long visit each time. There have also been times when I have not gone for three days because we are visiting one of my daughters or something else is going on.

She went through one of her phases recently, which lasted a few weeks, where she was very upset and even antagonistic toward me and probably everyone else. I would talk with her for a while, and she would tense up and scream, "Just stop!" I didn't know what to do, so I stopped. I didn't stay much longer.

During the last two or three weeks, she has been much more sedate and calm, except when an alarm goes off. The doors at the facility have alarms to alert the staff when somebody goes outside or just opens the door. There are also alarms on each patient to let the staff know if they have tried to get up or fallen out of their wheelchairs or their beds. For some reason, the alarm frightens my mom, and she thinks there is a fire or the police want her to go outside so they can arrest her.

Yesterday (the day before I am writing this), I went to visit her, and she was doing alright until the door alarm went off. She went into panic mode and was crying and very scared. I told her what I usually tell her: "Breathe deep, Mom." She did it, and it didn't help very well.

I then took the chance in doing something that sometimes helps and sometimes makes it worse. I grabbed her hand to hold it. Sometimes she doesn't want to be touched at all. But that day, she calmed down and started to gently rub my hand. It was a beautiful experience. I imagined it reminded her of me when I was a baby, and she would take my hand in hers and caress it. I will never forget yesterday; I don't think. Of course, one never knows what they will forget.

Sometimes she can answer some questions I have but not very often. That is also a glimpse into her "self" that I enjoy. I really enjoy especially when we can talk about my dad or her parents or when we were little. There is so much I don't know about her.

I must take the opportunities I have on her good days to find out interesting and helpful things about her and her family that I never knew. May God show me when these days come.

CHAPTER 4

What I Learned about
the State of Oregon

My dad was a very good father and husband. He was very busy earning a living, but when he spent time with us, he was fun to be around. When he retired and we were moved away, he loved to be with our families.

He worked very hard to earn a living so we could eat, live in a moderately nice house, and go to Christian schools. He even went to bat for my brother to get him on complete Social Security Disability. He did what he had to.

My dad also built a nice home in Northern California for himself and my mom during retirement. He had set up a retirement to set my mom for life, he thought.

They enjoyed living in their house and doing things retired people do. They went out to eat quite often and went on small trips and even long ones to visit their sons, wives, and grandchildren. It all worked out well until my dad passed away.

My mom was a reader, and she read that you should not make a move after your spouse dies until at least a year passes by. After that year and considerable conversation, we decided to move to a new location, and my mom would move near us. We were living in Northeast Washington at the time, and the winters were much too cold and severe for her. So we decided to move to Southwest Oregon in the Roseburg area.

It went really well for many years. She lived about eight minutes away from us. Rod also came to live with her. She had him for company when he was awake and out of his room. He had become somewhat of a recluse and slept strange hours.

After Rod moved into the nursing home, my mom felt like she should get out from under the strain of owning her house. She really worried about the upkeep of the house and yard and paid a lot of money to take care of them. She sold the house and moved into a retirement village where she really enjoyed all the social life, which she had not had much of after my dad passed away. My dad was her means of transportation. We took her to church almost every week, and at times, we took her out to eat and other things, but mostly, she was at home by herself. She never complained, but when she moved into the retirement village, she came alive socially, and we saw that she had missed that.

As mentioned before, my mom was always generous with her money after my dad passed away. She would help my brother Tim and I financially at times. She loved to do that.

The big time of giving came in the last three years. My brother's daughter got married, and she gave them money to help make it special, and we had sold our place and moved. We were looking for a country place and were looking for about three years before we found one. It was a good price, and we purchased it with the intension of remodeling it. It was absolutely unlivable.

It seemed like the remodeling would be within our budget, but a house needing to be remodeled is appropriately called a "money pit." We had to keep getting help from my mom. We were planning on having her live with us, and she was very happy to help us out.

I am ashamed to say how much over budget we were so I won't. Suffice it to say, it was quite a bit of money.

About six months before it was possible to live in the home, my mom had to go into a memory care facility. I got a free legal consultation about what I needed to do legally and financially to facilitate everything involved with the care of my mother. She had quite a bit of money at the time, so I didn't really worry about it. However, one thing the consultant said stuck in the back of my mind like a knife. I recently started to play with the knife to find out more about it. The knife was indeed sharp and painful.

In Oregon, if a person needs medical care and he or she drops down to $2,000 or below, they can go onto Medicaid. It seems great. But there are many different hidden problems about it. I will not go into all of them here, but everyone needs to look into it carefully.

They will not take your house into account to look at you going below the $2,000 threshold. However, if you are the surviving spouse or a single person, they will take what they have paid for out of your house after you pass away. It is possible that your descendants will get nothing out of it. This is what I was told by somebody I trust who knows what happens.

My mom doesn't own a home anymore, so it will not be a problem. I believe the Lord led in her decision to sell her home even though she lost some money on it.

The catch-22 that we are experiencing has turned out to be a much greater challenge, at least for us. If we had known, we would have done things differently for sure.

When the State of Oregon is seeing if you qualify for Medicaid, they look at how much money the person has. If they qualify that way, they look into the gifts given by the person applying. They ask for bank statements and go back five years to determine how much was given to family and/or friends. Basically, it seems as if the state of Oregon assumes that any gift of money (not sure if money is all they look at) was given for the purpose of defrauding the state. In order for the person to get down to $2,000, the ones given gifts must pay the amount back to the giver, and then the giver must legally spend that money down to $2,000. The state wants everyone to think that they help people so much, but many are probably living under adverse conditions because they don't have the care they need. Their family members, who are not properly trained in the appropriate care, have to take care of them, or they hire others to care for them who are not appropriately trained. They can't afford any better.

Now I will get into our situation.

At the time of writing this, my mom will most likely run out of funds by around the end of the year. If we wait until then, it could be a tremendous financial burden on our whole family, including my brother Tim's family. We can possibly take care of her with just the help of her Social Security and hopefully something from the military. But that probably won't cover food, supplies, gas for trips to doctors, and other caregivers to let Livi rest or recuperate from back pain. Our whole family would probably have to pitch in. We have not really discussed that yet. I hope we never have to have that discussion. I can work a little more, but likely have to also be home to help with my mom.

It really behooves us to make a decision soon—before she runs out of money. It will still be very hard. Livi and I have some plans for this year that might have to be cancelled also.

I am telling our plight so that others can avoid it. Please look into these things early on before you think you need to.

Since the majority of the money was given in the last three years, we have to go through three and a half years more to get past the five years. By the time anyone reads this book, the situation will be over because I don't plan on publishing it until my mom passes away—that is if I can get it published.

Another thing to know about is what you can expect from the Veteran's Administration. The VA does not tell anybody what they are eligible for. Apparently, a widow of a person who served in the military is eligible for some kind of pension and health insurance benefits.

I have been trying to get an appointment at the Veteran's Services office for over a week now. I have e-mailed them and gotten some response which leads me to believe that my mom qualifies for at least the pension. I also left a phone message, and they tell you not to leave multiple messages, so here I wait. Tomorrow, I will go down to the Veteran's Services office and try to get a walk-in appointment to apply for both unless I get a phone call or e-mail telling me of an appointment before then. I hope I have everything I need in case I can talk with somebody.

It is amazing just how unfriendly and difficult this world can be. A person really has to go into every situation armed with information, or you will be unsuccessful.

I am very thankful for the friend who happened to tell me of these benefits from the VA.

CHAPTER 5

A Made-Up Christmas Letter

In the first month of 2019, I decided to communicate with my mom's friends and family to let them know how she was doing but mostly to try to prime the pump for letters to be written to my mom. I knew that my mom would not and could not write the letter, so I made up what I thought she might write to let others know how she feels about things. This might be an idea others could use to help your loved one feel in touch with the outside world.

To My Dear Family and Friends:

I desire to wish you all a very Merry Christmas even though I am very late. You have been in my heart always even though I could not have you on my mind very often. I had a good Christmas. Jeff took me to his house, and I ate with him, Livi, Janet (their daughter), and Blake (her husband). I also got to talk with and see Tim and Linda on WhatsApp. We had a very good dinner. Jeff showed me a yearbook from Montebello High where I had attended and graduated from. I enjoyed that.

I have been getting progressively worse in my dementia. I sometimes can say things that make sense and are interesting to others, but it is not very often. I feel bad that I am rarely able to add anything to any conversation. It makes me very anxious that I cannot express how I feel. In fact, I cannot really know how I feel either. Sometimes I get very irritable and show it to others. I hate that I often express it toward my son and even his wife, Livi. Sometimes I can tell them that I love them very much. That makes me somewhat happy. I really never feel truly happy because of this disease.

I often cry and am very anxious and scared. When somebody asks me why I am anxious, I really do not know and I say that. Everybody seems to ask me the same questions all the time: How are you today? Are you feeling okay? Are you in pain? Do you have to use the restroom? What have you done today? I can hardly ever answer their questions.

A few times, when Jeff was visiting me and I was crying, my cry turned into a song. Once it was "For Those Tears I Died." Recently I hummed "Daisy, Daisy." I like doing that. It shows my family that I still know how to have a good time even though it is not that good. It also shows that I have the Holy Spirit still working on my heart.

I long to communicate, but I cannot do it very well any more. I used to be able to keep the communication open with all of you, but I can't anymore. So I have to do it through Jeff. But I can't tell him what to say, so he just keeps you informed about my life. It is embarrassing, but he feels you need to be informed because he covets your prayers and wants you to continue to send cards and letters. I really like to get them. I can remember you all even though my mind is very foggy. I also love you all very much, and thank you for being my friends and family who care for me.

God bless you all and Merry Christmas—any time is appropriate to speak of Jesus.

Ruby Bell

CHAPTER 6

Duty Seems to Be Obvious

Recently, I have noticed that my mom sometimes seems to be unimpressed with my visits. It seems like she believes I am visiting her out of duty and not out of love. Sometimes that is the case. It was especially the case lately when I had to move her to another facility, take care of transferring her prescriptions to another pharmacy, and spend many hours to try to get her help from the VA.

I have found that thinking of all these duties is not something you can turn off and on easily. I have only found two things that will help me. It is exactly what helps me in my morning worship to get my mind off of the cares of the day that are before me. I have to allot myself enough time for the visit with my mom and Jesus to not be behind when I am finished with the visit. I also have to pray that the Holy Spirit will "take these things hence" that take my mind away from the visit. When your mind wanders, bring it back.

I heard an interview with the photographer of Donald Trump's campaign. He said that Mr. Trump has the amazing ability to keep focused on the conversation he is having with a person even if somebody else enters the room that is more important or that he needs to talk with. Even if he is extremely busy, he can focus on talking with people and making them know that they are important to him. Certainly, my mom is very important to me. I don't want her to ever feel like she is not an important part of my life or that she is in the way.

CHAPTER 7

God Sometimes Has to Use Our Mindset

We often get into a mindset that it is hard to get out of. I do accounting. I am careful not to say that I am an accountant in general because that would limit what people think about me. However, I have worked on accounting for almost forty years with other types of jobs thrown into the mix.

As a person who does accounting, my mindset is often of a financial nature. I have the financial responsibility for my mom and take that responsibility very seriously. Being of that mindset, I might not notice other needs. But I have found out that I don't have to worry about that because God can use that mindset to get me to make decisions that the reasons for doing them are totally unrelated to finances. That happened to me about two months ago.

As I stated a few chapters ago, I noticed that my mom was running out of money, and she would no longer be able to afford to live in the memory care facility in the not-too-distant future. I was forced to try to find another solution. Part of that solution was applying for a pension for my mom from the VA. As I also mentioned a few chapters back, I was going to try to get a walk-in appointment to see about getting started on applying. The people at the Veteran's Services office were very nice and helpful. I found out they were not employees of the VA but were employees and volunteers of an agency that tries to help people get help from the VA. After several trips, I have my application finished and am just waiting to hear if they need any more information or if my mom will be getting some help. I am praying for the latter, of course.

Part two of the solution was to find another place for my mom to live. God made a way of escape that I knew not of. Antonina, who we have known for several years now, along with her husband, Daniel, owns and runs an adult foster home in a very beautiful location. I called her, and she miraculously had a place for my mom.

Livi and I went to see the place, and we were greatly impressed with the beauty and the atmosphere in general. The other residents are not screaming and carrying on like at the other facilities where my mom had lived. This is nothing against those other facilities but merely comes with the territory. With fewer residents, there are fewer disturbances.

Antonina has young children who live and play around the residents. My mom is in a family atmosphere, and it is really helping her. Antonina's little girl is only about fourteen months old (at the time of writing this) and is extremely sweet and cute. I saw my mom with a big smile for the first time in over a year and a half. She was smiling at little Sarah.

My mom is in a much better place now, and she is responding wonderfully. If you saw her, you would not think she is normal most of the time, but if you had a loved one that had the same problem as my mom, you would notice that she is improving. She communicates more and doesn't cry or moan nearly as much. I have also not ever seen her getting frustrated and lashing out emotionally at people like she had at the other facilities.

I want to point out again that I am not blaming the last facility. She got great care there. The whole thing is environmental. There are many people, however, who need the greater structure and security of the institutional-type facility.

The purpose of this chapter is to point out that God used my mindset of financial concerns to bring about a better environment for my mom. I cannot thank Him enough for circumventing my thinking. God is really love. We can cast all our cares upon Him, for He cares for us.

As time progressed, I was impressed to ask my mom's doctor to lower some of her meds and, maybe eventually, to get rid of some altogether. He was quite happy to lower one of her medications to see how it would result and to let him know in a month if we think he should lower it even more. It is so important to have a good geriatrics doctor who will work with you as the age of your loved one increases.

We actually were able to take my mom to a restaurant for Mother's Day which we would never ever venture to think about before she moved to the new place. It went really well, and she thanked my wife and me for the dinner. We also went sightseeing before the dinner in a beautiful rural neighborhood in Roseburg, Oregon, where the adult foster home is. She really only got anxious when we were on the freeway, which I figured was because it was too fast for her. I went on side roads taking her back.

All this improvement was only a side effect of my thinking. God indeed used my mindset to benefit my mom.

CHAPTER 8

Information Filter

It seems I am always wrestling with exactly what my mom should know about and what it is that is better for her not to think about. I have learned from trial and error as I see her overreact to news I have told her. Sometimes she can take things that other times she reacts badly to. Therefore, I not only have to figure out what she needs to know but also figure out her mood.

For an example, sometimes in the past, I have told her about working very hard mowing the lawn or cutting the blackberry vines or digging dirt to make the backyard level in order to be able to use the riding lawnmower in more places. At times, she has made a face like it has made her sad that I had to work so hard. At other times, she has taken it in stride. After all, I have to have something to say. I don't have a really exciting life. There are a lot of things happening but not much to write home about.

I have an idea that a relative has passed away, but it is not something I would ponder with her. That would make her upset for maybe nothing.

There was a time when she worked very hard on our genealogy and was very excited about it. She would try to talk about it with me and my brothers, and none of us were really into it, but we acted interested. Actually, I liked to look at the pictures and imagine myself back then in their life. However, I was far from being as interested in it as she was.

That was then, but now it makes her anxious to talk about it. It didn't take me too long to figure out why it made her so. To her, it is a big job still hanging over her head. In her mind, she has never finished that responsibility to her parents and family. In fact, when a person is limited on the responsibilities they can handle, they will still feel responsible for those things no matter how many times you tell them that they don't have to worry about those things anymore. It is not hard to see this. It could happen to any of us. We have unfinished goals, work, and plans. It is so sad. I have seen it in other people besides my mom. It was different with my dad. When he was in a coma, my mom said that I was taking care of things at their home. He formed the word on his lips, "*Good.*"

One very difficult thing to ponder if I should tell my mom about is what is happening in the lives of her friends and relatives. She no longer has an impact in their lives and some of them have told me they don't really want to see my mom in her present state. They would rather remember her the way she was. I can fully understand this. It is a hard thing to see someone who just sits there or makes little whining noises most of the time. Although my mom is much better at this time, she still has those strange habits and hallucinations some of the time. It is not very comfortable to talk with her when she just sits there during her "special" moments. And most people can probably tell that it makes her uncomfortable as well. So if I tell her that some people she knows are coming to visit us and they don't come to see her, I don't really know what to do. I can understand both situations.

CHAPTER 9

Is This a Miracle?

For the last four months, as I have been praying, I have been claiming the promise for my mom, "Be not conformed to this world: but be ye transformed by the renewing of your mind…" (Romans 12:2). I believe that God is able to do whatever is His desire for His people, and just maybe, it is His desire that my mom's mind be reclaimed.

I have seen a marked improvement ever since my mom moved to the adult foster care home. Now she is much better able to communicate and is somewhat like her old self. She has told Livi that she is very thankful for all we have been doing for her. Oh, how that makes us feel good because we went a couple of years not knowing if anything was doing her any good. That is when you have to trust that what God leads you to do is the best for her.

There was an interesting occurrence that happened one warm day when I took my mom outside on the balcony to look at the river and to read a devotional book to her. As I said before, I had been claiming Romans 12:2 every day for the renewing of my mom's mind. Well, the text for that day was Romans 12:2. It nearly brought tears to my eyes as I took it as a surety that my mom would pretty much recover her mind.

Of course, when you take God at His word, you wonder if you should tell others you expect more or if you have already seen the miracle. I believed that I had seen a partial miracle, and I was extremely thankful for that. It was difficult when I told my brother or my children that my mom was much better and when they saw her, she would have a bad day, or maybe what I was bragging about was not even near what I led them to expect.

Life became a little more normal. We started to take her out to eat which, as I mentioned earlier, was something we wouldn't dare do up to one month earlier. She seemed pretty calm and was able to enjoy herself to a point. I took her for more car rides than I had before, which was something she had always enjoyed before the disease. She used to love when she went with my dad for long rides looking at beautiful scenery. The scenery around here is indeed beautiful. The Roseburg area is in the beautiful Land of Umpqua. I wish I had taken her for a lot of rides when she didn't yet have the disease. I feel guilty that I spent the majority of my time working at my place and seeing her more out of obligation; although, I did enjoy the times I visited her.

But, even with the improvement, there was something still missing that was needed to make her be back to normal. The thing that was missing was consistency. God knows a lot about that because most of us are not consistent with our faith in Jesus. We are strong sometimes and then do something that shows we are very weak. My mom could carry on a pretty good conversation but then drift away into a different world. Even her conversations were a little bit skewed, and she would go back into her guilty syndrome far too often. My expectations were often dashed as I saw the hard reality of her disease.

I believe God is all-powerful, but it was His will that I sometimes had a problem with. Was this really leading up to an absolute miracle? Why wasn't the miracle I had already seen enough? I would have to wait and see.

CHAPTER 10

Can You Reach the Stage When You Are No Longer Useful?

Last Sunday, my wife and daughter and I took my mom out to eat at a local restaurant for her birthday, which was really the day before her birthday. We had a good celebration and gave her a couple of gifts. We all enjoyed it, but you would not know that my mom enjoyed it because she didn't really talk during the meal. She was too busy concentrating on getting the food onto her fork and to her mouth. She spilled on herself a few times and didn't appear to even notice it. Later that day, when I dropped my mom off, she thanked me and told me she had a wonderful time.

How could it be that she had a wonderful time when she barely entered into the conversation? I know she was not lying to me, but what we saw did not seem to match with what she said.

After thinking about it for a while, I figured out that at her stage in life, she needs to concentrate on the little things to coordinate herself. My mom was never one to talk very much when we had company, at least for the last fifteen years. However, she really enjoyed listening to everyone else having fun by joining in the conversation.

Two days later, in the morning, God showed me something truly amazing. My thoughts were that, after seeing my mom spill on herself and really concentrating on eating, she had passed beyond her usefulness in this world. That is not to say that she is not valuable to those who love her. I love her so much.

Then the Lord taught me that she might be more useful now than ever before. The way that she is causes us all to reflect on our own lives and attitudes and our relations with our fellow man. If the Lord tarries, we will all end up in a similar condition. Are we going to have loved ones around who will care for us? Are we going to care for others and not be self-centered at that time?

Most of us hope we will just die and not get into that condition. There is a descriptive word that people in that condition lose. That word is dignity. We have to have God's love for these people. Is it just my mom that I have to have this love for? Everyone is important.

Then the real tears flowed when I realized that our Lord and Savior allowed Himself to get into a similar situation as my mom. His dignity was completely taken away when He went to the cross. He was stripped at least almost naked. He was writhing in pain in front of hundreds of people. He most likely was stained by His own body functions (I hope I was led to express this in a reverent way). He was humiliated before the universe.

But He was happy to lay down His life because that was the only way He could save those who put Him on the cross. Let us lower our picture of ourselves because we are nothing compared to Jesus. Yet He values us as equal with Himself. Oh, what love.

It was like a progression of thoughts during that time of prayer because then I remembered that Jesus said unless we become as little children, we will not enter the kingdom of heaven. Little children dribble food all over themselves. They mess all over themselves and need to be cleaned up and changed. They spit up on their clothes. It doesn't cause them any concern. They are not embarrassed in the least. That is one of our greatest fears that we have. If we go to the bathroom and get our clothes a little bit wet or stained, we think, *How can I go out of the bathroom like this?*

> It was not enough that Jesus should die in order to fully meet the demands of the broken law, but he died a shameful death. The prophet gives to the world his words, "I hid not my face from shame and spitting."
>
> In consideration of this, can men have one particle of exaltation? As they trace down the life and sufferings and humiliation of Christ, can they lift their proud heads as though they were to bear no trials, no shame, no humiliation? I say to the followers of Christ, Look to Calvary, and blush for shame at your self-important ideas. All this humiliation of the Majesty of heaven was for guilty, condemned man. He went lower and lower in his humiliation, until there were no lower depths that he could reach in order to lift man up from his moral defilement. All this was for you who are striving for the supremacy—striving for human praise, for human exaltation; you who are afraid you will not receive all that deference, that respect from

human minds, that you think is your due. (E.
G. White: Review and Herald, July 5, 1887)

We need to get to the point where we can handle our greatest humiliation and think it is okay because we are only pointing to Jesus and not to ourselves. It is Jesus we need to make look good, not us—Jesus, precious Jesus.

I believe I have discovered the answer to whether or not we can reach the stage when we are no longer useful. The answer is a decisive *no*. Even after we die, our lives are still a testimony for good or for evil.

CHAPTER 11

The Disease Gets Bad Again

Around the end of August or first of September, we went through an experience similar to two years prior. My mom was starting to get very anxious again. Nothing seemed to be miraculous anymore. My hopes were falling apart. I heard from the caregivers Brenda and Denny (who took over for Antonina and Daniel while they were on an extended vacation) that my mom was more normal when I was not there, and when I came, she became very anxious. Brenda was doing everything she could to pray with my mom and calm her fears. She was even getting my mom involved in praying for the other residents in the home having her own ministry.

Yes, the disease was coming back. I was still praying but very alarmed. To top things off, my mom's finances were being drained. As I had done before, I came up with a new plan to use less of her money. That plan, this time, was to take care of her at home. My mom was not nearly out of money, but if we kept her at the adult foster care home, she would run out of money the early part of the next year. Since I had no idea how long my mom would live, I had to make provision for her money to last past the middle of the next year at least. Of course, I was still waiting to hear about the VA pension. We planned to bring my mom home on the twelfth of December, and we gave our notice to the Adult Foster Home.

In the first part of November, something happened that would change our plans. My mom went into ER on the fifth of November. I remember that date because it is my wife's birthday and our anniversary.

My mom did not really wake up that morning. She was taken to the breakfast table but was virtually nonresponsive. She was asleep almost all the time. The visiting nurse, who was not even visiting my mom, thought my mom might have had a stroke. She was taken to ER, and I got there as soon as possible with my wife following shortly after.

The ER doctors ran some tests, and they were inconclusive for stroke. The doctor told us that she might have had one or more ministrokes that don't show up on the CT Scan. They sent her back to the adult foster care home, and I kissed her goodbye, not knowing if she would get better. She was still basically nonresponsive.

Livi and I went to a restaurant to celebrate our special day, but our hearts were not really into it. We had my mom on our minds.

My mom improved the next day, but on the following Monday, she was back in the ER with the same condition. This time, it seemed much worse. We decided to have her stay in the hospital until we could arrange for her to come home. We needed to really get busy arranging a hospital bed, caregivers, and hospice. We were not giving up on her, but we wanted her to have some quality of life. To be honest, I really thought she would improve but was also realistic and wanted to provide good care in case it was the end.

She stayed four days in the hospital, and she came home to our house on Friday. Although the Adult Foster Home was a good situation, it was not the same as the care we could give her as a family. We had only one person to take care of and bathe with more love and attention (although the adult foster home caregivers provided a lot of both).

Cheri, a long-time family friend of ours really showed a lot of compassion for us and my mom. She offered to send us the money for two brand new chests of drawers to put my mom's clothes and toiletry supplies in. We will ever be indebted to her. She showed us the compassion of our Savior, and we praise God for her.

The trip home for my mom was exhausting, and she slept most of the time that day. While Livi was at work, we had a caregiver here at the house. I am not well versed in caregiving and could not handle it except for maybe an hour or so at a time. We had a separate caregiver for the weekend (if needed) and on Tuesday.

The next day, my mom was very alert in the morning, and Livi and the caregiver got my mom up, and she ate breakfast, and we set her in a chair and let her watch Christian music videos. I know she appreciated that but also slept most of the time, even getting up to the table was a little much for her. Her legs were not working well, and it took two people to transfer her. It might be that she actually had a few ministrokes that didn't show up on the CT Scan or maybe lying in bed for four days weakened her legs. Either way, she never recovered the strength in her legs. She stayed in bed the rest of the time.

When my brother, Tim, came, my mom was so happy. She had both of her boys with her. I knew that she was holding out until Tim got there. She ate and drank before he got there and while he was there in order to keep her strength up so she could spend time with him. Tim and I really enjoyed the time with her as well. We sang old songs we had written a long time ago, joked around, kissed her and basically tried to make it a family again, even though it was just us three left. Tim was there for about four full days, and we had a heartfelt goodbye.

My mom was ready to die after that because she basically quit drinking and eating the next day. I will leave a lot of blanks in this story for now because in the next chapter, I will cover a lot of it as well as some duplication. The next chapter will be much of my eulogy that I read at the memorial service. What a privilege that was to do her eulogy. It was also a privilege to care for her during her final days.

CHAPTER 12

The Eulogy

Although there is some duplication, I am excluding much of my eulogy for my mom at her memorial on December 15, 2019. All that is pertinent to my family and my mom's friends is not necessary for everyone to know, and I want to try to include those things that would be helpful to others facing similar situations with their loved ones as well as items that make it more interesting, at least in my opinion.

I was very pleased to have all the family there. My brother Tim, his wife, Linda, their oldest daughter, Melissa, her husband, John, and their youngest daughter, Stephanie, all came to share in the honor. My oldest daughter, Janet, her husband, Blake, my youngest daughter, Crystal and her husband, Michael, as well as our grandchildren, Benjamin, Mia, and Katelyn were also there. Of course, Livi was there as well.

Eulogy for Ruby Bell (Mom)

To our family, my mom was like the recording angel. She had a record of all the events in our lives. She wrote a lot down, but she remembered much of it anyway. She knew more about us than we did ourselves. I knew that when she passed away, I was in trouble. She had written the eulogies for my dad and my brother. Who would write it for her? My memory about those things is not very good, and the memory of my younger brother, Tim, is even worse. He claims he can't remember anything if it happened more than six months ago. My older brother, Rod, had a great memory. At one time, he thought maybe he could remember things that happened when he was in the womb. But he's not available to help either.

What was I to do? Well, the Lord knew what to do. As I was pouring over my mom's many genealogy books that were carefully organized to have a few pictures in each book to make it harder for me to gather them, I happened upon a few pages that were titled "My Life's Recollections." Lo and behold, my mom came through again as the recording angel. Although it was only the first twenty-two years of her life, it was enough to make the story of her life interesting. I was to be born three years later, so maybe I could remember a lot of what happened in her life, maybe.

I think I figured out why my mom remembered so much about all of her family's lives. I believe it is because she prayed so much about every aspect of our lives. She also got involved if we let her. I remember she actually read my accounting book over winter vacation. I couldn't imagine anyone doing that if they didn't have to. Later in life, when I was working, my mom would love to just sit at the kitchen table and watch me eat supper hoping I would say something about my day. My mom cared about us.

Here goes the eulogy:

Ruby Bell was born in 1932 in Montebello, California, to Charles and Pearl Bohn. She was their only child, but she had three half siblings. Her father was a widower when he married my grandma. He was quite the entrepreneur. He owned a few businesses including a used car lot. He was not your typical stereo-typed used car salesman because he was honest.

He was also very helpful and generous as I gleaned from the notice of his death in his church's newsletter. (It was important to me to find these things out because I never met my grandfather and always wondered what kind of a man he was. He died when my mom was only twelve years old.)

As a youth, she mostly did things with the church youth. She met my dad, Jess Bell, about the time she graduated from Montebello High in 1949. They started going out that Christmas Eve. They both enjoyed going places with their friends from church, and they liked to sing together. My mom would play the piano. They got engaged before my dad got drafted into the army. They were married April 25, 1951.

My dad was a second lieutenant in the army. He got shipped out to Korea in September of 1952. That was one of the saddest days of my mom's life.

My mom loved to travel on family vacations, and she always took care of all of us unselfishly. We took vacations every summer—sometimes to family and sometimes just to enjoy places we had never seen. We lived in Baldwin Park, California, from when Tim was only a newborn to when he was about thirty. My parents then moved to Magalia, California, to a home my dad had built. They really enjoyed life there in their country place. My mom loved when any of us would visit. My mom worried quite a bit about the fact that there were no good escape routes in the case of a fire. That came true a year or so ago when the fires destroyed Paradise, California, and much of Magalia. I never told my mom about it because I knew she would worry about her friends and even her beautiful house, which was destroyed. She was living a life of dementia at the time.

The last two weeks of her life I did a lot of looking at her face. In the hospital, she was asleep most of the time, and so I could only see her face. She finally woke up and was amazingly different. When she was awake, she actually communicated much like old times. After we brought her home, she was a changed woman. She was in a weakened condition, but when awake, she was happy to be at our place. When Tim came, and she saw him for the first time, she had a big glorious smile on her face for a long time. She did a lot of smiling at both of us as we talked with her and each other. She always loved to hear us talk and laugh together. Livi and the other caregivers did a wonderful job of making her comfortable. While I am on the subject, I want to thank all the caregivers who cared for my mom when she was at Chantele's and especially when at Rainbow's End and at our home. They exemplified compassion.

The time Tim was with us was very fulfilling. I am forever grateful for him coming and for God arranging it. It was very sad when he left because we all knew it would be the last time he would ever see her on this earth. The very next day, she started eating and drinking almost nothing. And the day after that, she didn't eat or drink anything.

She continued like that until Wednesday morning when she breathed her last. I believe God woke me up that morning to notice her breathing differently. I got Livi up, and she said, "This is it. All we can do now is pray with her and let her know we are here and that she has nothing to worry about."

I never got tired of seeing her face. Even after she passed away, I kept staring at her face knowing it would be the last time I would see her before Jesus returns. I am so glad I was able to serve my mom up to her last breath. One might think of it as an obligation, but I saw it as a privilege. I know Livi did as well and

Tim too. Now I only have Tim left, and I am very happy I do. We both know we need each other.

This time with my mom also confirmed my need of Jesus Christ. I don't know how I could have handled it without Him. It is time to get right with Him. We will need to hang on to Him as the times get harder, and you have nowhere else to turn. Thank you, Jesus. When that happens, many will finally realize what a gift our Savior is.

My mom's life ended in November, but I still feel I can serve her by serving Jesus. In fact, I feel like I am serving her by honoring her here today. She was a great woman. The text that comes to mind when I think of my mom is Isaiah 42:3: "A bruised reed shall he not break, and the smoking flax shall he not quench." She never intentionally hurt anyone in my whole life. She cared for everyone she knew.

Of course, the verse refers to Jesus, and He is our example in all things, but it is good to have some everyday people examples as well. I believe my mom was one.

I am so thankful that God finally answered my prayers. I often prayed that my mom would stop being tortured by Satan and that I could have some indication that the Holy Spirit was getting through to her. Well, I saw that during her last days. Oftentimes, God uses one's death to stop the devil's attacks. But God gave us all a gift. He stopped the attacks early this time.

CHAPTER 13

Tying Up Some Loose Ends

One of the purposes of this book was to be informative. But, mainly, I wanted it to be helpful. I wanted anyone going through the experiences I have to know what they might expect. This chapter is all informative—telling you what you might expect when you lose a loved one. It is certainly not exhaustive. However, I believe I have given enough examples to be very helpful to anyone reading it.

VA

As I mentioned in chapter 7, I got a lot of help from VA Services. I got a very good caseworker who was very helpful, and I thought I might just get help for my mom—a pension. I had no idea how much it would be, but I had hoped that it would prolong the time before my mom ran out of money.

After many times of meeting with the caseworker and having to give the same information over and over in a different format, we had to make the decision to bring my mom home to stay with us. We hadn't heard from the VA. As I mentioned before, it was sped up by her final illness. Then when she passed away, I wrote an e-mail to my caseworker telling her that I guess

I would not get anything. I was very upset that the VA wasted a tremendous amount of my time.

After I sent that e-mail, the caseworker thought the case might be far enough along so we could possibly get the money owed to my mom when she was alive. The VA even acknowledged my request and sent me more forms to fill out. Finally, I got a letter from them telling me that I would get nothing unless I was a dependent child of my mom's or her surviving spouse. The caseworker at VA Services told me that was the end. There is indeed at least a lot of incompetency in that organization.

During the many times I have waited at VA Services to be helped, I have heard many horror stories about veterans who have spent many years fighting with the VA to get the medical help they need and deserve. I feel sorry for them all.

Health insurance

Before my mom's death, I was like a bull behind the gate at a rodeo. I was just waiting for her death to go crazy and try to accomplish everything I needed to accomplish and get it over.

One of the first things I did was to call her insurance company to cancel her insurances. She had her supplemental medical insurance and her prescription drug plan through the same organization. I made one call telling them my mom had passed away, and the insurance had to be canceled. Now that was over—I thought.

On my mom's next month's bank statement, I saw that her supplemental insurance was still being charged. I called to let them know, and they said I never called to cancel it. I vehemently told them that I had called. In fact, it was the day my mom passed away. Then they let me know what they should have told me when I called: that you have to let both legs of insurance (medical and prescription drug) know.

If I ever get into this situation again, I will know. But there was no way to know when I called the first time because they didn't tell me.

Social Security

I quickly found out that the Social Security Administration cannot keep the next payment from coming. I had to have my mom's bank cancel the payment and send it back. Maybe if you give them enough notice, they can do it. But I could not have given them any more notice. I called them on the same day my mom passed away. So you need to be prepared that there will probably be a payment that has to be sent back.

My mom's bank account

If you are the power of attorney on your loved one's bank account, the moment that person passes away, you are no longer the power of attorney. The paperwork has to be changed to have yourself be the main signer on the account. You have to get an EIN (Employee Identification Number) for the account and use that instead of the loved one's social security number or yours.

That was the only thing I needed a lawyer for in the whole process of executing the distribution of my mom's assets.

Life insurance paperwork

Well-before your loved one is close to dying, you need to investigate any life insurance policies you can find. I found out that the original company (my dad got the policy in the 1960s) had been bought out at least twice. I had a very difficult time tracking down the company.

Not only was it difficult investigating but it was also difficult finding out if the policy was still in effect. This is because they would not talk to me or answer any questions until I proved to them that I had the power of attorney. This, in itself, was a very difficult thing to do. I think the whole process took about a month.

Even after the death, there was difficulty. The company sent a form that I had to have notarized that said I and my two brothers were the only children my mom had. I had to have a witness that knew that for a fact. All my witnesses I could use are nowhere near here. I called the company with my concern. They told me just to get a neighbor and go before a notary with her as a witness even though my neighbor had no idea if we were the only ones. It worked.

A somewhat humorous thing happened when we went to the bank to get the form notarized. The lady commented, "You don't have Rodney's address." I exclaimed, "He's dead!" She said, "Oh, that's right."

Grave plot lure

My parents bought a couple of grave plots in the veterans' section of a cemetery in Southern California. Since then, my dad decided he wanted to be cremated and wanted his remains placed in my mom's arms in the casket and buried in one of the plots. The other plot they wanted for Rod. Well, my mom also decided she wanted to be cremated, and Rod also was cremated.

The best thing to do was that my mom would sell the two plots. However, nobody thought of that until after my mom got the dementia and could not handle her own business. Tim called the cemetery and found out that a burial plot is not like any other property. The children of the owner(s) cannot sell the plots until the owner(s) are gone even if they have power of attorney.

We also found out that what they purchased was almost worthless because it was only the plots. Another $1,500 or so per plot would still have to be paid in order to bury your loved one there. There's an opening and closing fee, a permit charge, and who knows what else. In my opinion, these cemeteries rip people off because they don't make things clear about all the extra charges. I know my dad would never have purchased these things if he knew everything was not paid in full.

When I went to inquire about burying my dad, brother, and mom in the cemetery almost across the street from our place, I learned from the mortuary that any cemetery owned by a large corporation would gouge people. It would take around $2,000 or more to buy one plot and put all three urns in it. It might be even more because they also charge a fee for each urn. That doesn't even include a gravestone.

The mortuary suggested I use another cemetery nearby that was not owned by a large corporation. I got the plot for about $250, and it was opened and closed for only about $350. If I chose, I could have dug it up and closed it myself for free. I even got a very nice gravestone for all of them that will be placed soon.

Get burial insurance

I would suggest to anyone to get burial insurance. The social worker for my brother told me it was one of the best purchases for my brother to get his funds down under $2,000. It was a very good piece of advice.

Everything was paid for in the case of my brother. In the case of my mom, we even got money back because originally we had planned to have my mom's body shipped to Southern California and buried in one of the grave plots as was the original wish of my dad.

Tax-free inheritance

I have learned that in Oregon, you do not have to pay income taxes for the first $1 million of inheritance. You don't have to pay federal taxes for the first $5 million. That was very good news to me, and I am sure to most of my readers.

Notice of death in newspaper for any of your loved one's creditors

I was told I might have to place a notice of my mom's death in the newspaper for about three months in order to give a chance for any of my mom's creditors to have an opportunity to collect anything belonging to them. That made me more stressed than anything else I had to do after my mom's death because I was afraid it was just an opportunity for scammers to claim my mom owed them lots of money.

I was very happy to learn from the funeral director that most people don't do that. It is really to be done when your loved one was behind in his or her bills. However, I would still suggest that you enquire what the law is in your state.

Final tax return

A final tax return (IRS Form 1041) is required if the estate or the deceased person generated more than $600 of income in their last year of life.

Trustee reimbursement

In Oregon, the maximum amount a trustee can get for their services in distributing the assets of the estate is 3 percent of the total value of the estate when it is between $10,000 and $50,000 and 2 percent when it is above $50,000. A professional can charge whatever is the going rate. You need to check the laws in your state.

Death certificates

It is important not to order too many death certificates. A lot of places will accept a copy of one or will need an original but can send it back after they have received it. I have always ordered too many. I could have probably gotten by with just ordering four or five (or maybe even less).

Did a relative pass away

In section 2, chapter 8, I mentioned that I had a feeling that a relative of my mom's had passed away. Well, after my mom passed away, a notice I sent to a relative came back, and her phone number was no longer a working number. I looked on the internet and discovered that she had passed away in October 2018. I also found out that my mom's best friend from her youth passed away the same month and year. Death is all around, isn't it?

Can't tell my mom anymore

Now it has been ten months since my mom has passed away. I can't tell you how often I think that I need to share something with my mom and I cannot—some things only she would appreciate. I just have to live with the reality of the situation. I will just share everything with the Lord who appreciates all the information my mom would.

The flip side is also true. I can't ask my mom anything anymore either. Many things I could have known if I had my mom to ask are now buried with her. I am sure there is information that nobody can know anymore unless God decides to share it. Perhaps many things are better not known.

God's timing

So many things have happened since my mom passed away. The Lord's timing is wonderful. With the COVID-19 pandemic, my mom would have been even more scared and would not have understood why nobody ever came to visit her. People are not allowed to visit their loved ones in a facility anymore. My mom and we were spared that situation, thank God. And right now, we are experiencing terrible fires in Western Oregon. My wife and I have had to evacuate. However, the Lord has caused the fire to be stalled, and it looks like our house will survive. The weather should turn even more in our favor in the next few days. We are moving back into our house tomorrow. My mom was terribly afraid of fires. Her death might not have been as peaceful in these times. We thank God for His timing.

A SHORT EPILOGUE

I pray that this book has been really helpful to anyone who has not been through this type of experience yet and for anyone wrestling with some of these issues currently.

People need help in navigating the pitfalls of pain and suffering during the sickness and death of a loved one. I also felt like getting these thoughts out on paper in order to better think things through for myself.

My faith in Jesus Christ came out in my rethinking as I knew it would. Jesus is a big part of my life, and going through these things makes you thankful for this tremendous Friend.

Thank you for taking the time to read this short book that was put together with much concern for my fellow human beings. I wish I had read a book like this before I went through this experience. But I probably would not have been interested in it–thinking it could never happen to me or my family.

ABOUT THE AUTHOR

Jeff Bell was born and raised in Southern California. He got his bachelor's degree in business management from Loma Linda University. He worked for three years and returned to Loma Linda to get his MBA. He worked in an ad agency for three years and quit to pray and read the Bible to get right with Jesus. After about four months, he eased back into work as part-time accountant for a private school and continued while working other accounting jobs through a temp agency until he married Livi Maldonado and started a new life in another area. They have two daughters who they love very much.

After marrying, Jeff has had many jobs in accounting and office management. His family moved to Oregon and then Washington where he worked for several small businesses and met the challenges of straightening out their accounting. He moved back to Oregon to be near his mom after his dad passed away. At the time of this writing, he's the part-time accountant for a small ministry.

Being handicapped, Jeff has insight into life that few have. He has gone through trying times increasing his ability to discover things in his life and the lives of others. He is very self-analyzing, as you will see from the book. He loves to help others, which is the main purpose of this book. He's sent out the chapter entitled "Can You Reach the Stage When You Are No Longer Useful?" and has had wonderful responses thanking him for the helpful words, especially from those caring for their feeble loved ones. That indicated to him that the book needed to be published. He hopes to help you, as the reader, and encourage you to really appreciate your loved ones while they're still around.